Hamza KHALED

All about Ruminant Q fever

Hamza KHALED

All about Ruminant Q fever

and relationship with human disease

ScienciaScripts

Imprint

Any brand names and product names mentioned in this book are subject to trademark, brand or patent protection and are trademarks or registered trademarks of their respective holders. The use of brand names, product names, common names, trade names, product descriptions etc. even without a particular marking in this work is in no way to be construed to mean that such names may be regarded as unrestricted in respect of trademark and brand protection legislation and could thus be used by anyone.

Cover image: www.ingimage.com

This book is a translation from the original published under ISBN 978-620-3-44017-1.

Publisher:
Sciencia Scripts
is a trademark of
Dodo Books Indian Ocean Ltd. and OmniScriptum S.R.L Publishing group
Str. Armeneasca 28/1, office 1, Chisinau-2012, Republic of Moldova, Europe
Printed at: see last page
ISBN: 978-620-5-28010-2

PREAMBLE

This manuscript discusses the main aspects of animal Q fever, as well as the existing relationship with human disease, as it is a widely distributed zoonosis throughout the world.

It is intended for veterinarians, animal health technicians, breeders or any person having an activity related to agriculture and/or animal production and health. In addition, the general public could benefit from the information contained in this simplified document to facilitate the assimilation of its contents.

The ultimate goal of this initiative is the popularization of infectious diseases that affect both animals and humans. The example taken in this manuscript deals in an easy way with an infectious disease that is often very poorly known and neglected, since it is not routinely diagnosed either in animals or in human medicine. However, it has attracted more attention since the epidemic in the Netherlands, which caused a lot of damage to health and economy.

TABLE OF CONTENTS

<u>INTRODUCTION</u>

Reproductive disorders are one of the most serious scourges in animal production; those caused by infectious diseases occupy an important place, among them *Coxiella burnetii*, a bacterium with obligatory intracellular multiplication, agent of Q fever, a disease widely reported throughout the world, resulting in abortions, stillbirths or weakened newborns, infertility, placental retentions and metritis, thus causing considerable economic losses.

In humans, the endemic nature of the disease, its severity, and the reported epidemics confirm that Q fever is an important public health problem. The social impact of the disease is closely related to the populations in rural areas and some urban areas with specific conditions.

Nowadays, there is a considerable lack of epidemiological information, both in animal and human health. This state of affairs does not allow an accurate estimation of the incidence of Q fever in animals.

Across different countries, very few studies have been carried out and are essentially limited to serological surveys in certain regions; in addition, the absence of a specific surveillance system for this disease makes it very difficult to objectively assess its importance.

CHAPTER 1
HISTORY

In 1937, Q fever was first described by EDWARD DERRICK, who was contacted about a febrile illness that was occurring among slaughterhouse personnel in BRISBANE, AUSTRALIA, in 1935. When cultures and serological tests failed to reveal a diagnosis, DERRICK suspected a new disease. He carefully described the characteristic clinic and named the disease "Q fever" (fever of unknown origin). He demonstrated that it was possible to transmit the disease to laboratory animals by inoculation with the blood of humans suffering from acute Q fever.

Although DERRICK initially concluded that the infectious agent was a virus, the study completed by MACFARLANE BURNET in MELBOURNE indicated that the pathogen was a Rickettsiae, in the terminology used at the time.

However, DERRICK might not have been the first to transfer the disease to laboratory animals. Another researcher named HIDEYO NOGUCHI who worked at the ROCKEFELLER Institute in NEW YORK in 1925, passed *C. burnetii* to guinea pigs from ticks that had been collected at MONTANA. Nevertheless, this microbial agent, was eventually lost after several passages in laboratory animals.

Around the same time that surveys were being made in AUSTRALIA, GORDON DAVIS was studying Rocky Mountain Purple Fever. He observed that a febrile disease originated from ticks collected around the vicinity of NINE MILE CREEK. This disease produced did not resemble Rocky Mountain Purple Fever. Subsequently, HERALD COX was able to characterize the organism (then called the Nine Mile agent) as similar to the rickettsiae and cultured it in the yolk sac of the embryonated chicken egg, he named it *Rickettsia diaporica.*

The relationship between Q fever and the Nine Mile agent was established by ROLLA DYER in 1938, in an event that foreshadowed the problems of Q fever transmission among laboratory workers, himself acquiring acute Q fever.

DERRICK proposed the taxon *Rickettsia burnetii* in 1948, and CORNELIUS PHILIP proposed that this bacterium be considered the only species in this genus different from other Rickettsiae. The causative agent of Q fever was finally designated *Coxiella burnetii* in homage to both COX and BURNET following the isolation and characterization of this new pathogen.

Following the clinical description and microbiological characterization of the etiology, the disease has been identified in at least 51 countries on 5 continents.

A first detailed analysis of more than 560 scientific publications was published in 1959 by BABUDIERI.

Q fever has had many synonyms, the most commonly used are: Coxiellosis; Balkan influenza; OLYMPUS fever; 7-day fever; CRETE pneumonia; DERRICK and BURNET disease; NINE MILE CREEK fever.

CHAPTER 2
EPIDEMIOLOGY OF Q FEVER

2.1. Frequency and geographical distribution

The difficulty of knowing Q fever and its estimation is a problem raised internationally. Recently, researchers have started to look for the real prevalence of the disease, as most of the previous works had completely different objectives. They aimed to measure the degree of involvement of the disease in reproductive disorders, as well as the study of the different routes of elimination of the germ in the external environment. Since inapparent forms are very frequent, this contributes to the underestimation of the importance of the prevalence in livestock.

2.1.1. In ruminants

In animal Q fever, knowledge is limited, perhaps due to the controversial reliability of its diagnosis, especially the complexity of animal epidemiology and the multitude of possible transmission routes. Currently, Q fever in ruminants is the subject of much research, due to its proven involvement in human outbreaks, especially in small ruminants.

2.1.2. In humans

Human Q fever has been reported throughout the world except for NEW ZEALAND and the ANTARCTIC region and many epidemiological investigations are trying to find the link between human infection and that of domestic and wild animals.

In sub-Saharan Africa, the clinical manifestations of Q fever in children are similar to malaria. In areas where malaria is endemic, most fevers are attributed to *Plasmodium falciparum* and consequently, children undergo expensive treatment.

In EUROPE, we are witnessing an increase in the incidence of the disease and the number of epidemics, among the most affected countries, we can mention :

- **THE NETHERLANDS:** Since 2007, several waves of human cases have occurred, constituting the largest episode of Q fever in humans ever reported internationally, with 982 and 2305 confirmed cases in 2008 and 2009. The incriminated goat herds have been subject to increasingly drastic measures.

- **FRANCE:** The frequency of the disease is not precisely known because Q fever is not a notifiable disease. From non-epidemic seroepidemiologic studies, the attack rate was estimated at 1 case/1000 inhabitants/year. A serological survey among blood donors recorded a prevalence of 4.1% (38 cases out of 924 individuals tested).

- **GERMANY:** A recent study reviewed 40 epidemics between 1947 and 1999. The authors note that these outbreaks are increasingly urban. 24 outbreaks were sheep-related, 6 outbreaks were cattle-related, the 2 oldest outbreaks occurred in research laboratories, while for 8 outbreaks no source could be suspected.

However, the prevalence rates recorded across the African continent are serious:

- **ALGERIA:** Overall seroprevalence has been estimated at 18.5%, ranging from 7.7% in urban areas to 35% in rural areas. An earlier study found a rate of 15% among slaughterhouse workers in Algiers and 20% among children under 16 years of age in the Hoggar region.

- **TUNISIA:** 26% seroprevalence has been recorded across the country. In the central-eastern part of the country, 55 cases have been confirmed over 10 years.

- **MOROCCO:** A rate of 1% was reported in the west and 18.3% in the central region.
- **MAURITANIA:** A 33% achievement rate was recorded.

2.2. Biological Reservoir

The study of the epidemiology of *Coxiella burnetii* in animals is complicated because most animals, especially ruminants, have been found to be seropositive for this bacterium when tested.

A wide variety of animals can be infected with *C. burnetii*: horses; dromedaries; pigs; rabbits; mice and other rodents; buffaloes; primates; reptiles; amphibians; domestic (chickens; pigeons; turkeys; ducks and geese) and wild birds; fish and marsupials.

In addition, dogs and cats may account for some of the Q fever cases in urban areas. Recently, *C. burnetii* has been isolated from marine mammals, from seal placenta.

2.3 Methods of transmission

2.3.1. In animals

a. Respiratory tract

Most cases of Q fever result from inhalation of contaminated aerosols or dust from parturients or slaughtered ruminants.

A placenta infected with *Coxiella burnetii* left outdoors can infect herds several kilometers away.

b. Digestive tract

Oral contamination of ruminants occurs as a result of ingestion of feed contaminated with parturition products, but it is not considered an important route.

c. By insects

Transmission of *Coxiella burnetii* by ticks is also possible. There are more than 40 species of ticks that are naturally infected with the bacterium since they can ingest it during their blood meals. Therefore, the excreta of infected ticks are considered a possible source of transmission because the microbial load can be high.

Flies also play a significant role in the transmission of Q fever, especially mechanical transmission.

Among the incriminated species are: *Musca domestica*; *Melophagus ovinus* and *Stomoxys calcitrans*.

d. Venereal route

Coxiella burnetii can be isolated from semen, but sexual transmission of infection, if possible, does not play a major role in the epidemiology of this disease because it is much less efficient in disseminating the infectious agent than excretion at the time of abortion.

e. Embryo transfer

Recent studies have demonstrated the presence of *Coxiella burnetii in the* zona pellucida of goat and cattle embryos, which may implicate embryo transfer in the transmission of the bacterium between infected donor females and healthy females and their offspring.

2.3.2. In humans

a. Respiratory tract

The most common route of infection with *Coxiella burnetii* is the respiratory route. The disease appears after inhalation of aerosols from slaughtered animals or parturient women, in farms, slaughterhouses, or even in laboratories where these animals or their organs have been studied.

Aerosols can be derived from infected fluids such as delivery fluids, urine, feces and milk.

Another probability of transmission is related to the inhalation of tick feces if they contain a significant load of bacteria.

b. Digestive tract

Ingestion of contaminated raw milk leads to positive seroconversion and not to clinical manifestations of Q fever.

c. Other ways

There are more routes that are classified as minor in the transmission of human Q fever, these include:

- the fetomaternal route in pregnant women;
- tick bite;
- blood transfusion;
- direct from person to person or after autopsy;
- kidney, bone or heart transplants;
- sexual contact.

2.4. Propagation

2.4.1. Transhumance

The fact of having attended a transhumance represents a factor of dissemination of *Coxiella burnetii*, several epidemics confirm it, one can quote:

- **SWITZERLAND**: in the VAL DE BAGNES, in 1983, 415 cases were diagnosed after a transhumance of 900 sheep.
- **ITALY**: in 1996, in the region of VICENZA, the investigation highlighted the role of flocks of sheep that had crossed the area of the epidemic, 53 cases were confirmed.

- **FRANCE**: in 2002, in the CHAMONIX VALLEY, where the disease was linked to contact with sheep or to a transhumance, the number of cases was 89.

2.4.2. Wind

The role of wind in the dissemination of *Coxiella burnetii* has been well elucidated, thus explaining cases of disease not related to animal contact. It is estimated that the pathogen can travel up to 40km. The best known example is the 1989 epidemic in England, 147 confirmed cases of Q fever were linked to the spread of the wind from a rural area to an urban area.

CHAPTER 3
CLINIC

3.1 In ruminants

Theoretically, the clinical manifestations of Q fever in infected animals depend on several elements: species; age; sex; host immune status; bacterial strain; inoculum dose; and route of transmission.

Few clinical manifestations are associated with animal Q fever. The disease is responsible for reproductive disorders in cattle, sheep and goats: late abortions; stillbirths or weakened newborns; infertility; placental retention and metritis.

When the bacterium first comes into contact with a herd, a wave of abortions is observed in pregnant females, then the enzootic evolves periodically and the number of abortions decreases. Overall, abortions are more frequent in small ruminants than in cattle; in the latter, the disease can still cause pneumonia, which can affect a significant proportion of the herd and would precede the abortive episode when it exists, followed by infertility and more rarely metritis. However, enzootic abortions have been much more frequent in goats where early abortions are the exception. Placental retentions are rare, but more common in goats and cows.

Regarding lesions associated with abortions, the placenta becomes edematous and sometimes autolyzed, with normal appearance of the cotyledons. The intercotyledonary areas may be edematous and thickened, sometimes with a yellowish exudate. Microscopically, placentitis, placental vasculitis and even thrombosis may be observed. The immune response during Q fever is associated with an inflammatory reaction that leads to the formation of granulomatous lesions most often involving the lungs, liver and bone marrow. Although the histologic lesions are nonspecific, *Coxiella burnetii* induces granulomas in affected organs centered by a lipid vacuole with a fibrinoid corona. As for the abortus, it is often normal, but because of the delay between fetal death and abortion, it may sometimes be autolyzed or mummified. In some cases, liver congestion may be seen.

3.2 In humans

Coxiella burnetii infection is asymptomatic in about 50% of cases, otherwise it manifests itself in acute or chronic forms.

a. Acute form

The incubation period varies from 2 to 3 weeks, with extremes of 4 days to 6 weeks. Acute Q fever usually evolves in 3 forms:

- **Flu-like syndrome:** involves a very high fièvre, of abrupt onset and may be associated with headache, asthenia, and myalgias. The fièvre may last long enough to be considered a prolonged fièvre of undetermined origin.
- **pneumonia:** most cases are mild with a non-productive cough and minimal auscultatory abnormalities. Pleural effusion or even acute respiratory distress may be associated.
- **Hepatitis:** with hepatomegaly sometimes painful but rarely icterus, these manifestations are associated with an increase in serum transaminases.

Because its symptoms are nonspecific and variable, the diagnosis is often missed. Cases of bone marrow necrosis, lymphoadenopathy, diarrhea, hemolytic anemia, febrile rash, myocarditis, pericarditis, phlebitis and meningoencephalitis have been reported. In addition, the disease can be responsible in pregnant women for abortions or recurrent miscarriages.

b. Chronic form

Endocarditis is present in 60-70% of cases. The chronic form can occur from one month to several years after the acute form, or even in the absence of a history of this form. Occasionally, the disease can cause osteomyelitis, hepatitis and prolonged fever.

c. Long-term sequelae

A set of symptoms has been reported under the name "Chronic Fatigue Syndrome":

- inappropriate fatigue;
- night sweat;
- myalgia;
- arthralgia;
- mood swings;
- sleep interruption;
- loss of libido.

CHAPTER 4
BACTERIOLOGY

4.1. Systematic

Phylogenetic studies based on sequencing of the 16S rRNA subunit have shown some relatedness between *Coxiella burnetii* with the genera *Legionella*, *Francisella* and *Rikettsiella*. Currently, it is classified in :

- **phylum:** *Gammaproteobacteria* ;
- **order:** *Legionellales* ;
- **family :** *Coxiellaceae* ;
- **genus :** *Coxiella*
- **species:** *C. burnetii* (only species present).

4.2 Morphological characteristics

Coxiella bumetii is an obligate intracellular bacterium. They are small pleomorphic cocci (0.4 to 1μm long and 0.2 to 0.4μm wide).

Their surface is composed of 3 membranes resembling those of Gram-negative bacteria since it contains :

- an external membrane, very rich in lipopolysaccharide (LPS) and proteins;
- peptidoglycan;
- an internal membrane.

C. burnetii has a gene similar to the one found in *Escherichia coli* that is responsible for capsule production, suggesting that this bacterium may possess this ability under certain circumstances.

<u>**4.3 Genetics**</u>

<u>**4.3.1 Genome**</u>

The genome of *Coxiella burnetii* is composed of a circular chromosome of 1.5 to 2.4 Mb and a facultative plasmid of 36 to 42 Kb whose function is still undetermined. The size of the genome is variable between different strains.

The movement of *IS* gene elements was involved in the genomic plasticity of *C. burnetii* with the presence of 83 pseudogenes. DNA-DNA hybridization studies showed that the strains are homogeneous and the genetic variation in this bacterium is of geographical origin.

The percentage of G+C is equal to 42 to 43%.

<u>**4.3.2. Plasmid**</u>

Some strains possess plasmids, but it is not yet proven that they code for certain virulence factors. Although plasmids were present only in some strains of *Coxiella burnetii* isolated from human cases of endocarditis and abortions in goats. In contrast, other plasmids were only present in acute infections.

The plasmids isolated to date are:

- **QpH$_1$** : isolated from the Nine Mile strain, its size is 36 Kb ;
- **QpR$_s$** : isolated from the Prescilla strain, its size is 39 Kb ;
- **QpDG:** the 51 Kb one was isolated from the Dugway strain and the 40 Kb one from the chronic Q fever cases;
- **QpDV: there are** 2 of them, one with a size of 33,5 Kb and the other with 56 Kb.

<u>**4.4 Development cycle**</u>

There are 3 cell forms in *Coxiella burnetii* that are associated with different stages of the development cycle:

- **Large Cell Variant (LCV): it is** a variant with large cells, (0.2µm wide and 1 to 2µm long), it represents the infectious form of the bacteria. It is found in the intracellular compartment and multiplies to give other LCV, or the 2 other forms.
- **Small Cell Variant (SCV): this is** a metabolically inactive cell, with a size of 0.2µm wide and 0.5µm long. It represents the form of resistance and persistent infection in the host.
- **Small Dense Cell (SDC):** called pseudo-spore, it represents the precursor of the extracellular form. It is a compact variant of small size (0.4µm wide by 0.7µm long), which constitutes the extreme form of resistance of the bacteria, found inside the infected cell or in the external environment.

SCV develops from LCV as a result of asymmetric cell division. It is distinguished from LCV by its regular rod shape, a thick layer of peptidoglycan and proteins between the two layers of the cell envelope, with a condensed nucleoid.

LCVs are much more polymorphic, have scattered and granular nucleoids or sometimes fibrils in their cytoplasm.

Nucleoid condensation or dispersion may be associated with the presence of small 20 kDa proteins that bind to DNA. A number of proteins, which are differentially expressed in SCV and LCV have been described. ScvA and HQ1 are specific SCV proteins that are localized in the cytoplasm. These proteins are thought to have structural roles in the formation of the condensed nucleoid of the SCV form.

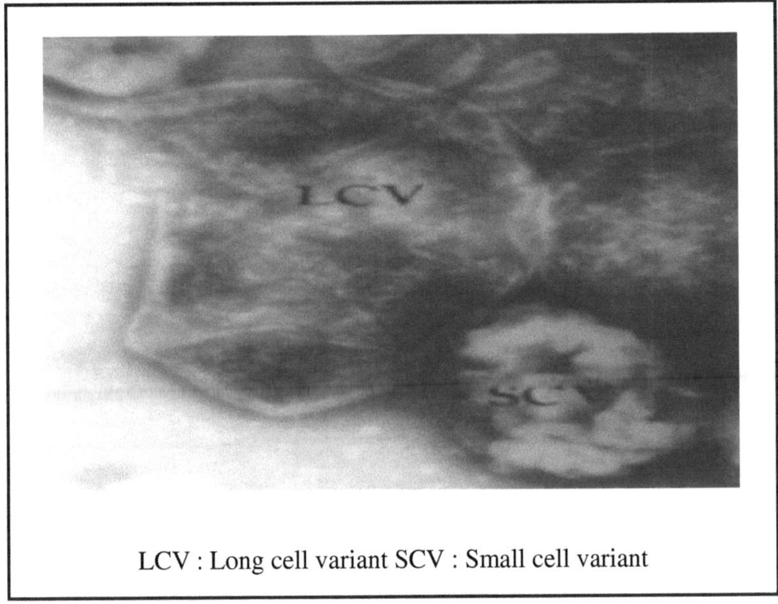

LCV : Long cell variant SCV : Small cell variant

Figure 1: Developmental forms of *Coxiella burnetii* by electron microscopy

4.5. Antigenic characteristics

4.5.1. Phase variation

Repeated passages in cell cultures or embryonated eggs produce attenuated rough or phase II strains from virulent or phase I strains of *Coxiella burnetii*. This phenomenon is comparable to that observed in *Enterobacteriaceae*. It is a mutation in the genes coding for the enzymes that synthesize LPS. Phase II has the property of multiplying rapidly *in vitro*, but *in vivo* it is sensitive to complement activity. However, phase I is the infectious form found in nature, the conformation of its LPS makes the bacterium resistant *in vivo to the* action of complement by the absence of the fixation of the C3b fraction, and thus blocking the access of antibodies to the bacterial surface.

4.5.2. Antigenic constituents

a. O-chain: it represents the dominant antigen of the immune response. The LPS of *Coxiella burnetii* in phase I contains sugars that are absent in phase II, these sugars have been identified as L-virinose (6-deoxy-3-C-methyl-gulose), dihydrohydroxystreptose (3-C-hydroxymethyl-pentose) and galactosaminuronyl-α(1,6)-glucosamine

On the other hand, the LPS of *C. burnetii* in phase II contains only 2 sugars which are D-mannose and D-glycero-D-manno-heptose.

b. Lipid A: it contains much more acyl chain (16-C) relative to other Gram-negative bacteria.

4.5.3. Antigenic communities

Coxiella burnetii has antigenic communities with :

- *Bartonella henselae*;
- *Bartonella quintana*;
- *Chlamydia trachomatis*;
- *Chlamydia pneumonia*;
- *Chlamydia psittaci.*

4.6. Culture

Initially, *Coxiella burnetii was* cultured in the yolk sacs of embryonated chicken eggs.

Subsequently, several types of cell cultures were put into use, the most known are :

- **Vero**: epithelial cells of African green monkey kidney;
- **BHK-21**: hamster kidney fibroblast;
- **L-929**: murine fibroblast ;
- **HEL**: human embryo lung fibroblast ;
- **HeLa**: epithelial cells of a human cervical carcinoma ;
- **CHO**: Chinese hamster ovary fibroblast.

The germ culture is relatively slow and the generation time is never less than 8 hours. The slow growth of *C. burnetii* is thought to be a reflection of the single rRNA operon copy, since the presence of low copy numbers of the rRNA operon is a trend in slow growing bacteria, including other obligate intracellular bacteria.

4.7. Metabolism

Coxiella burnetii is characterized by an acidophilic metabolism, because most of its transport mechanisms required for the acquisition of necessary nutrients from the vacuoles will function in a pH range of 3.0 to 5.0.

a. Carbohydrate metabolism

C. burnetii is able to utilize glucose, probably by the EMBDEN MEYERHOF-PARNAS oxidative pathway. However, the lack of enzymes in the initial pathway (glucokinase or the phosphotransferase system that can convert glucose to glucose-6-phosphate) is replaced by a carbamoyl phosphate-dependent trans-phosphorylation of glucose.

b. Amino acid metabolism

C. burnetii is characterized by a strong auxotrophy towards several amino acids. The uptake of extracellular amino acids and their precursors is probably mediated by a group of 13 transporters derived from the hydrolysis of protein complexes by lysosomal proteases and other enzymes secreted by *C. burnetii*.

c. Lipid metabolism

C. burnetii lacks MEP (2-C-methyl-D-erythritol 4-phosphate), a pathway for isoprenoid biosynthesis which is a common component of Gram-negative bacteria. This bacterium synthesizes 2 sterol reductases (CBU1158 and CBU1206) which are extremely rare in prokaryotes. Their probable role is the conversion of cholesterol precursors for the formation of the paracithophore vacuole (VP).

4.8. Resistance

a. Survival in the external environment

At +4°C, the viability of *Coxiella burnetii* is retained for 1 year or more in passive vectors such as dried tick feces, wool, and non-chlorinated water. The bacterium can persist for 5 months in soil and 4 months in dust. In foodstuffs, the bacterial survival is maintained more than 42 months at +4°C in milk, for meat, it remains infected for at least 1 month in a conservation temperature.

b. Resistance to physical agents

Compared to other cell-multiplying bacteria, *Coxiella burnetii* has a high resistance to environmental stresses such as: high or low temperature (down to -20°C); osmotic pressure (pH above 4.5) and ultraviolet light. Total inactivation is not always achieved by exposure to 63°C for 30 min, or 85-90 C° for a few seconds. Their destruction by gamma rays requires a dose of 6.6×10^5 rads. For sera, the dose must be equal to 5.5×10^6 rads.

c. Resistance to chemical agents

Coxiella burnetii is resistant to common disinfectants such as 0.5% formalin, 0.5% bleach, 5% hydrogen peroxide and 1% phenol. This bacterium is rapidly inactivated by diethyl ether, but not by ethanol. Also, it is resistant to formaldehyde used without humidity, but becomes sensitive when used with 80% humidity.

d. Antibiotic resistance

Bacteriostatic activity has been demonstrated for Nine Mile and Priscilla strains with doxycycline (10 mg/ml), rifampicin (1 mg/ml) and ofloxacin (10 mg/ml). However, L929 cell cultures are used to test the sensitivity of *Coxiella burnetii* to antibiotics.

CHAPTER 5

PATHOPHYSIOLOGY

5.1. Pathogenesis

The different stages of the *Coxiella burnetii* survival cycle are shown in Figure 2.

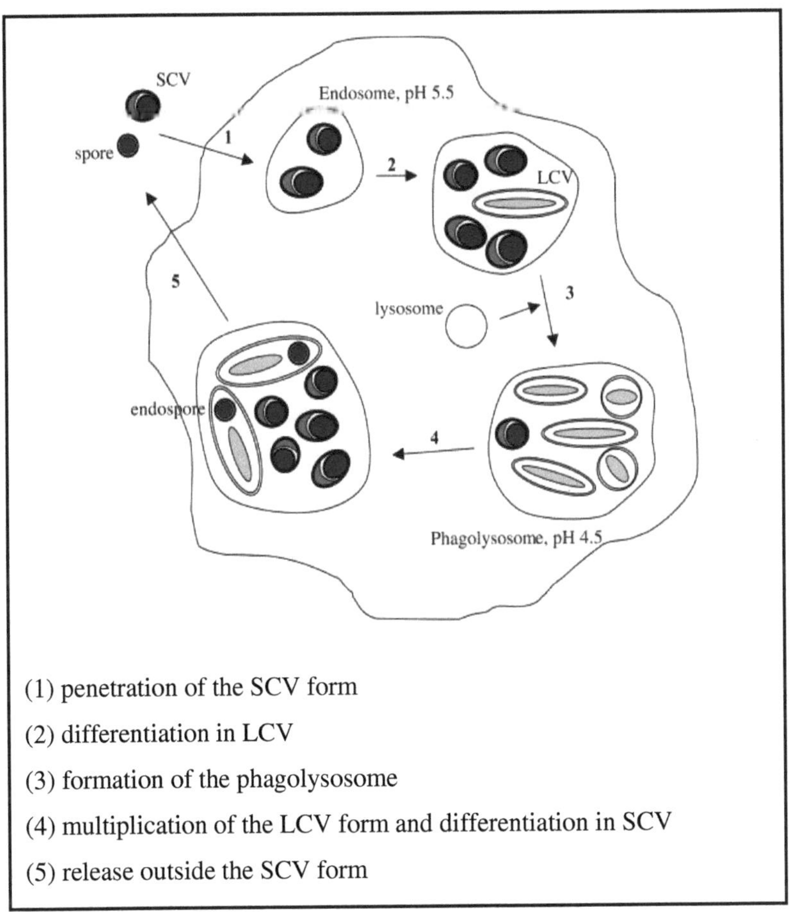

(1) penetration of the SCV form

(2) differentiation in LCV

(3) formation of the phagolysosome

(4) multiplication of the LCV form and differentiation in SCV

(5) release outside the SCV form

Figure 2: Development cycle of *Coxiella burnetii* in a **host** cell

a. Penetration

Infection of animals and humans occurs most often by the airborne route, in some cases by the digestive route, therefore the primary targets of the bacteria are alveolar macrophages in the lungs and Kupffer cells in the liver. However, the bacterium has actually been found in blood monocytes and macrophages in many other organs such as: spleen; bone marrow; pancreas; heart and other lymph nodes.

In female mammals, a peculiarity is found in the preferential localization of *C. burnetii in the* uterus and mammary glands. The adherence of the bacteria appears to be a passive phenomenon, since the inactivated bacteria penetrate with the same proportions as the living bacteria.

b. Internalization

After attachment of bacteria to cellular receptors that are specific according to the bacterial phase, their internalization into monocytes and macrophages occurs by endocytosis. Phase I bacteria interact with integrin $\alpha_v \beta_3$ while phase II bacteria involve integrin $\alpha_v \beta_3$ and the complement receptor CR3. However, other factors, such as hydrophobicity, would allow better internalization of phase II bacteria.

A reorganization of the actin cytoskeleton was observed after the interaction of phase I bacteria with their receptor, which will induce protrusions at the attachment site of the bacteria and thus, its internalization by endocytosis. Since this phenomenon was not observed in phase II bacteria, it could also explain the differences in the internalization rate of *C. burnetii* in the 2 phases.

c. Merger and multiplication

Once inside the cell, the phagosome containing the bacteria would fuse with the lysosomes and form a VP similar to a secondary lysosome. It is from this stage that SCVs will differentiate into LCVs. The multiplication of *C. burnetii* takes place in large numbers in the VPs which have the characteristics of phagolysosomes. Their pH around 5 activates the metabolism of the bacterium and initiates its replication. Subsequently, the phagosome, which is rich in LCVs, condenses into SCVs or initiates sporogenesis which results in the formation of SDC forms (also called pseudospores) and continues to interact with the autophagic and endosomal pathways of the cell. This form confers the properties of preservation and dissemination of the bacterium, found inside the infected cell or in extracellular condition, it is at the origin of most natural infections and is thus of crucial importance in sanitary prophylaxis.

C. burnetii has been shown to possess acid phosphatase activity which may explain its ability to inhibit the oxidative action of neutrophils. In addition, *C. burnetii* possesses superoxide dismutase, catalase and CbMip (macrophage infectivity potentiator) which provide protection against the microbicidal effects of reactive oxygen intermediates from host cells. In addition to these enzymes, two alkyl hydroperoxide reductases (AhpC and A hpD) play a protective role when the gene coding for catalase is inactive or truncated.

In vitro, exposure of *C. burnetii* to an acidic environment can trigger the synthesis of a number of proteins. This activation is thought to mirror the initial production of the proteins *in vivo* and therefore they represent a tool to study their importance for the early phase of infection. Among them are the heat shock proteins Hsp62 and Hsp71.

The average isoelectric point pI of proteins synthesized by *C. burnetii* is 8.25, of which 45% have a pI greater than or equal to 9, compared to other intracellular bacteria such as: *Mycobacterium tuberculosis*; *Brucella suis* and *Chlamydia trachomatis* with an average pI of 7.24 to 7.40. However, the expression of a high number of basic proteins would allow the bacteria to survive in the phagolysosome which represents a hostile environment for bacteria.

d. Pathophysiology of abortion

A strong bacterial multiplication has been observed, in trophoblastic cells, the week before abortion. This bacterial colonization of the placenta could trigger abortions, stillbirths, premature deliveries or the birth of stunted animals. These clinical observations have been reported especially in small ruminants and occasionally in cattle.

According to SIDI-BOUMEDINE et al, (2010), Q fever is considered the agent of abortion when the amount of bacteria is greater than or equal to 10^4 per vaginal swab.

5.2. Virulence factors

Very little is known about the genes responsible for the pathogenicity of *Coxiella burnetii*, but it is generally accepted that wall LPS plays an important role. Inoculation of guinea pigs with *C. burnetii* LPS is responsible for clinical and pathological changes similar to those observed with inoculation of live germs.

5.3. Infecting dose

It has been assumed that a single bacterium is capable of causing disease, but rather, it has been shown that a microbial load of 200 cells/m^3 in the air was necessary to establish an infection during an exposure time of 30 min to 1 hour.

5.4. Portage

In infected females, *Coxiella burnetii is* present in the placenta and fetal envelopes, after parturition, in milk during lactation, and in urine and feces.

Non-pregnant females are less susceptible than pregnant females. In goats, infection at mid-gestation causes the most abortions, while infection at the end of gestation results in the birth of live but infected offspring that may abort their first gestation, if female, or excrete bacteria in the semen if male.

However, there is no experimental study of the influence of gestation on susceptibility to infection in cattle and sheep

5.5. Excretion

The proportion of excreting animals is quite variable in infected herds and the kinetics of bacterial excretion by different routes would be irregular.

The germ is excreted in the milk, urine, feces and uterine discharges of infected ruminants. Bacteria are present in very high numbers in the amniotic fluid, placenta, and fetal membranes of parturient or aborted animals. These animals can continue to shed infectious particles long after abortion (10^9 bacteria per gram of placenta in goats after abortion and at least 70 days in ewes.

During 2 successive pregnancies, abortions and vaginal excretion of *C. burnetii* were observed in goats. In contrast, ewes aborted only once with Q fever.

Generally, females recover quickly after abortion. In cattle, no study to date has shown whether or not the bacterium disrupts several successive pregnancies as it does in women, goats and mice.

Infected dairy cows excrete bacteria into the milk for many months. The duration of the infection in dairy goats is not known, but may correspond to that of cows. The average in milk is variable from more than 15 days after delivery to several months (even more than 36 months).

There is no systematic link between the appearance of clinical signs and excretion in milk. *C. burnetii* was detected in sheep milk for more than 3 months after parturition. However, these initial results, which need to be confirmed, would seem to indicate that excretion in sheep milk is less frequent and persists for a shorter period of time than in cattle and goat flocks.

In cows and goats that have aborted, excretion is not systematic in the milk and, if it is the case, this excretion can be of short duration, contrary to other females of the herd that have apparently normal births and that will excrete for several months or even for several lactations.

However, fecal and vaginal excretion in sheep is very high and seems to persist longer than in milk.

In cases of metritis, this excretion seems to persist for a long time.

5.6 Immunity

5.6.1 Humoral-mediated immunity

The protective role of specific antibodies has been studied in animals and several experiments have concluded that the humoral response alone cannot control the multiplication of *Coxiella burnetii*. Throughout the infection, IgG antibodies against phase II are present. An IgM titer greater than 50 indicates acute Q fever or primary infection. In contrast, a high antiphase I antibody titre indicates a chronic form of the disease.

5.6.2 Cell-mediated immunity

Although the antibody response may be closely associated with the characteristics of the acute disease, cell-mediated immunity is most important in the definitive eradication of the bacteria and the prevention of chronic manifestations of infection.

The cells of the innate immune response are the first ones involved in the control of bacterial multiplication, during an infection or a vaccination. *In vitro*, macrophages infected by *Coxiella burnetii*, produce pro-inflammatory cytokines such as TNF-alpha, IL-1 alpha in the 3 hours post-infection. The production of these cytokines via the interaction of bacteria with the TLR2 receptor of macrophages would limit bacterial multiplication. The IL-12 cytokine would activate Th1 helper T lymphocytes which would induce the production of INF gamma which, in turn, would act on bacterial multiplication. However, for the infection to be eliminated, the infected monocytes are eliminated following the cell death signal delivered by TNF-alpha. During a *C. burnetii* infection, other interleukins are involved, such as IL-10, which is involved in the replication of *C. burnetii* and in the evolution towards chronicity by interfering with TNF production.

To maintain its niche, the bacterium is able to inhibit apoptosis by inhibiting the activation of caspase cascades and to increase the expression of anti-apoptotic proteins (A1/Bfl-1, c-IAP2).

Another survival mechanism has been linked to the maintenance in phosphorylated form of proteins involved in the cell survival signaling cascade, resulting in decreased apoptosis of host cells following infection.

5.7. Experimental pathogenicity

- **Guinea pigs:** The susceptibility of guinea pigs to *Coxiella burnetii* is variable. Adults respond better to infection. Intraperitoneal injection causes hyperthermia, after an incubation period of 5 to 12 days, lesions are observed in the spleen, liver, testicles, inguinal and mesenteric lymph nodes. Myocardial degeneration is frequently observed as well as pulmonary congestion.

- **Mice:** inoculation of mice by intra-nasal and intra-peritoneal route shows the presence of nodules at splenic, hepatic and renal level 4 to 6 days later.

- **Hamster:** this animal is particularly suitable for the study of this germ. After intraperitoneal inoculation, the bacteria are isolated from the spleen, high titers of antibodies are detected, even higher than those found with mice and guinea pigs.

- **Monkey:** to study human Q fever, the macaque represents the best study model. After 7 days of exposure, respiratory distress was noted with interstitial pneumonia and hepatitis.

CHAPTER 6
DIAGNOSIS

6.1. Direct diagnosis

6.1.1. Choice of sampling

In animals, specimens may be obtained from placenta, vaginal discharge, and the abortus (lung, liver, and stomach contents) just after abortion or parturition.

Milk (mixed or individual), colostrum and fecal samples can also be studied.

6.1.2 Isolation

Since all strains of *Coxiella burnetii* have a high degree of infectivity, they should be handled in a BSL-3 laboratory. Isolation can be done directly by inoculation of embryonated chicken eggs or by use of cell cultures.

6.1.3. Microscopic examination

Since they are alcohol-resistant bacteria, they can be stained by several methods: modified Ziehl-Neelsen, Stamp, GIMENEZ, GIEMSA or modified KOSTER stains. Their detection presumes the presence of the pathogen. Sometimes, bacteria can be difficult to detect because of their small size.

6.1.4 Immunohistochemistry

Immunohistochemistry can be used either on paraffin-embedded tissue or on acetone-fixed smears. It is an indirect immunofluorescent or enzyme immunoassay using polyclonal antibodies to *Coxiella burnetii*.

6.1.5. PCR

Only Polymerase Chain Reaction (PCR) can easily identify herds and animals shedding the bacteria. This technique has been the most important contribution to the diagnosis of Q fever in recent years and several kits are available using conventional PCR or real-time PCR (qPCR), single or multiplex.

Several genes or sequences have been used successfully in different types of samples, the most used are:

- *IS1111* gene and the *icd* gene;
- superoxide dismutase gene;
- isocitrate dehydrogenase gene ;
- rRNA sequences;
- outer membrane proteins com1 ;
- QpH1 and QpRS plasmids;
- htpAB heat shock proteins.

Indeed, recent data show that the number of the insertion sequence (*IS1111* which codes for transposase) varied considerably between 7 and 110 depending on the isolate. It is sufficiently informative for high quantities of bacteria (greater than 10^4 per vaginal swab) for the diagnosis of abortion.

PCR goes through several steps: initial denaturation of the DNA; denaturation; primer pairing (or hybridization) and elongation. Real-time PCR consists of monitoring the amplification process over time by means of fluorescence. The data of this fluorescence are collected at each cycle of the PCR and represent the quantity of amplified products at this moment. The emission is directly proportional to the amount of amplicons generated, the more concentrated the sample is in target molecules at the origin, the fewer cycles it will take to reach a point where the fluorescent signal is significantly higher than the background. This point is defined as the Ct (threshold cycle) and appears at the beginning of the exponential phase. This concept of Ct is the basis of the precision and reproducibility of the technique.

If we follow the fluorescence, thus the number of amplified PCR fragments, we distinguish 3 phases:

- **Background phase:** the amount of fragment amplified is insufficient to generate a fluorescent signal above the background.

- **Exponential phase:** the amount of amplified fragment generates a fluorescent signal above the detection threshold of the device, then the number of amplified products doubles at each cycle. This phase is represented by a straight line in logarithmic coordinates.

- **Saturation (plateau) phase:** certain components of the reaction (in particular the number of *Taq* polymerase molecules available) become limiting. The system no longer allows exponential amplification.

The experimentally obtained Ct values as a function of the log of the fixed target molecule concentrations are represented by a standard line from a series of dilutions of a known sample. The Ct value is inversely proportional to the log base 10 of the initial target concentration. From a sample of unknown concentration, the Ct obtained will be translated into concentration in target molecules thanks to the standard line.

The choice of effective and specific primers must respect several rules:

- **length:** in practice, the number of nucleotides is between 20 and 30 bases. Sequence: the sequences of the 2 primers of the same pair must present the maximum of divergences and more particularly at the 3' end, in order to avoid their Co-hybridization.

  The G+C content should be about 50%. GC richness improves the stability of the primer-matrix duplex.

- **concentration:** optimal concentrations for 30 cycles vary between 10 and 50 pmoles of each primer.

- **number of cycles:** to obtain a detectable signal on gel, 10 molecules must be amplified in 35 cycles under optimal conditions.

Too many cycles will result in the accumulation of non-specific products.

- **temperature:** the hybridization temperature is specific to a primer. It is calculated from its Td (dissociation temperature), temperature at which half of the duplexes formed are dissociated, several techniques are possible:
    - SUGGS formula: it applies only to perfect duplexes of 11 to 20 bases. For duplexes larger than 20 base pairs. $Td° = 4(G+C) + 2(A+T)$.
    - MCCONAUGHY formula: For hybrids with more than 20 base pairs:$Td° = 81.5-16.6(Log(Na+))+0.41(\%G-C)-(600/N)$. Where G and C represent the number of nucleotides and N is the number of bases in the primer.

6.2. Indirect diagnosis

Since the clinical diagnosis of Q fever is very difficult, the use of serology is an alternative.

The criteria to be considered for the judicious choice of a method are: sensitivity; specificity; positive predictive value; cost and choice of antigen.

Serological investigations have the major disadvantage of providing information on exposure to the germ, but they do not detect it. It is thus after 5 weeks of lambing that the antibody titers reach the maximum and that there are the most conversions and they persist several months.

In acute Q fever, anti-phase-II antibodies predominate and their titers exceed those of anti-phase-I. Like most infectious diseases, IgM antibodies are the first to appear.

6.2.1. Fixing the complement

The Complement Fixation (CF) method is very specific but lacks sensitivity. Lytic antibodies can persist for long periods after disease, in return, seroconversion is detected later compared to the Indirect Immuno Fluorescence (IFI) or Enzyme Linked Immuno Sorbent Assey (ELISA).
The appearance of false negatives in chronic disease is related to the prozone phenomenon.

6.2.2. ELISA

This technique has excellent sensitivity and specificity. In veterinary medicine, it is preferable to the complement fixation technique and immunofluorescence, it looks for anti-phase I and anti-phase II antibodies.
A seropositive herd is not necessarily a herd that excretes *C. burnetii*. The antibody response persists for at least 2 years, even in the absence of clinical signs and shedding.

6.2.3 Immunofluorescence

In human medicine, indirect immunofluorescence (IFI) is the gold standard for the serodiagnosis of Q fever. This technique looks for IgG, IgM and IgA immunoglobulins for phases I and II. Seroconversion is detectable 7 to 15 days after clinical onset. Immunoglobulin titers peak at 4 to 8 weeks and then decrease progressively over the following 12 months.

6.2.4 Intradermal reaction

A skin test method has been proposed to study the cellular response and to improve the detection of infected animals at the herd level. A nodule of variable size appears at the injection site if the animal has been previously infected with Q fever.

CHAPTER 7
TREATMENT AND PROPHYLAXIS

7.1. Treatment

7.1.1. In animals

In ruminants, antibiotic treatment usually consists of 2 injections of oxytetracycline (20 mg per kg body weight) during the last month of gestation, although this treatment will not completely suppress abortions and excretion of *C. burnetii* at lambing.

In known infected herds, administration of tetracycline (8mg/kg/day) prophylactically in the water supply prior to parturition may reduce the spread of the organism, although administration of antibiotics to treat or prevent Q fever is still a highly undesirable method.

7.1.2. In humans

Doxycycline 100 mg twice daily is recommended for acute forms. Co-trimoxazole is most commonly used in children under 8 years of age.

In addition to the recommended treatment, the new Macrolide molecules can be used.

To treat chronic Q fever, 18 months of treatment with Doxycycline (100mg twice daily) or Hydroxychlorochine (200mg, 3 times daily) seems sufficient.

7.2. Prophylaxis

7.2.1. In veterinary medicine

Prevention of animal Q fever is based on reducing or avoiding contact between the source of infection and susceptible species, and on stimulating host resistance through vaccination.

The identification of a Q fever free herd is particularly delicate. It can never be based on a single negative PCR analysis of the mixed milk, but must combine a serological analysis of about ten sera and several successive PCR analyses of the tank milk. The sera to be analyzed will be taken in privilege on females having had problems of reproduction.

7.2.1.1. Sanitary measures

Since the excretion of *Coxiella burnetii* reaches its maximum at the time of abortion or parturition, in addition to the very high infectivity of placentas, the general hygiene measures applied to placentas and manure are the most appropriate to implement, they correspond to :

- the farrowing in a specific box which must be disinfected;
- The manure must be treated, as well as the slurry which must still be neutralized with calcium cyanamide;
- destruction of placentas and aborted babies, by incineration, rendering or treatment with lime, in order to avoid their ingestion by domestic or wild carnivores. These measures should be applied away from the wind, which may spread the germ.
- administration of antibiotics such as oxytetracycline (20 mg/kg live weight) in the last month of gestation reduces the abortion rate as well as the excretion of bacteria at the time of delivery.

Defensive sanitary measures are aimed at limiting the introduction of the germ into flocks with a known favorable sanitary status and are based on :

- precautions when introducing or mixing animals (screening, quarantine and limiting the risk of contamination during transport, not introducing animals from herds of unknown health status);
- precaution with regard to neighbouring farms (better physical separation and limiting contact between animals);
- isolation of females at the end of gestation;
- prohibition of the loan of males between herds ;
- synchronization of pregnancies in small ruminants.

- precaution against other vectors of *C. burnetii*. In areas of high tick infestation, sanitary control measures should be adapted and vaccination is recommended.

7.2.1.2. Vaccination

Vaccination against Q fever has long been suggested for the prevention of human infection and to reduce economic losses at the farm level.

Several studies reveal a great deal of variation in the methods of vaccine manufacture, the strains of *Coxiella burnetii* and in which phase they are used, the nature of the adjuvants and the antigens used. Vaccines prepared from phase I strains show a significantly higher efficacy than those from phase II, the latter being less hazardous to handle.

COX-VAC (monovalent vaccine composed of *C. burnetii* antigens in phase I and CHLAMYVAX FQ (bivalent vaccine composed of *C. burnetii* in phase II and *Chlamydia abortus*) are effective vaccines and provide better protection against Q fever, combined with hygiene measures and other appropriate control plans for ruminants.

7.2.2. In human medicine

7.2.2.1. Sanitary measures

The measures to be recommended are not specific to Q fever. They are preventive measures common to all diseases that may occur in livestock and that may cause human contamination. They include restricting contact with animals during the calving period and providing hand washing facilities.

7.2.2.2. Vaccination

Vaccines prepared from phase I strains were 100 to 300 times more potent than phase II vaccines. However, they may cause induration at the injection site and granuloma formation. Currently, the most widely used vaccine is Q-Vax Phase I. It has proven to be more effective in protecting at-risk populations. Its protection lasts more than 5 years with 100% effectiveness in certain situations.

<u>BIBLIOGRAPHIC REFERENCES</u>

Agence Nationale de la Sécurité Sanitaire de l'Alimentation, de l'Environnement et du Travail (ANSES), "Fièvre Q: Rapport sur l'évaluation des risques pour la santé publique et des outils de gestion des risques en élevage de ruminants", Report adopted by the Expert Committee on Animal Health on June 8, 2004, (2004), 88 p.

Ayres, J.G., Smith, E.G. and Flint, N., "Protracted fatigue and debility after acute Q fever", The Lancet, V. 347, (1996), 978.

Berri, M., Laroucau, K. and Rodolakis, A., "The detection of *Coxiella burnetii* from ovine genital swabs, milk and fecal samples by the use of a single touchdown polymerase chain reaction", Veterinary Microbiology, V. 72, (2000), 285-293

Bildfell, R.J., Thomson, G.W., Haines, D.M., Macewen B.J. and Smart, N., "*Coxiella burnetii* infection is associated with placentitis in cases of bovine abortion", Journal of Veterinary Diagnostic Investigation, V.12, (2000), 419-425.

Cabassi, C.S., Taddei, S., Donofrio, G., Ghidini, F., Piancastelli, C., Flammini, C.F. and Cavirani, S., "Association between *Coxiella burnetii* seropositivity and abortion in dairy cattle of Northern Italy", New Microbiologica, V. 29, (2006), 211-214.

Cetinkaya, B., Kalender, H., Ertas, H.B., Muz, A., Arslan, N., Ongör, H. and Gurçay, M., "Seroprevalence of coxiellosis in cattle, sheep and people in the east of Turkey", Veterinary Record, V. 146, (2000), 131-136.

Coleman, S.A., Fischer, E.R., Howe, D. , Mead, D.J. and Heinzen, R.A., "Temporal analysis of *Coxiella burnetii* morphological differentiation", V. 186, no. 21, (2004), 7344-7352.

Dellacasagrande, J., Capo, C., Raoult, D. and mege, J.L., "IFN-gamma-mediated control of *Coxiella burnetii* survival in monocytes: the role of cell apoptosis and TNF," Journal of Immunology, V. 162, no. 2, (1999), 2259-2265.

European Center for Disease Prevention and Control (ECDC), "Panel with Representatives from the Netherlands, France, Germany, United Kingdom, United States of America. Risk assessment on Q fever", ECDC Technical Report, 40 p.

European Food Saftey Authority (EFSA), "Panel on Animal Health and Welfare (AHAW). Scientific opinion on Q Fever", EFSA Journal, V. 8, no. 5, (2010), 114p.

Fenollar, F., Fournier, P., Carrieri, M.P., Habib, G., Messana, T. and Raoult, D. "Risk factors and prevention of Q fever endocarditis", Clinical Infectious Diseases, V. 33, (2001), 312-316.

Guatteo, G., Seegers, H., Taurel, A.F., Joly, A. and Beaudeau, F., "Prevalence of *Coxiella burnetii* infection in domestic ruminants: A critical review", Veterinary Microbiology, V. 149, (2011), 1-16.

Ghigo, E., Capo, C., Raoult, D. and mege, J.L., "Interleukin-10 stimulates *Coxiella burnetii* replication in human monocytes through tumor necrosis factor down-modulation: role in microbicidal defect of Q fever", Infection and Immunity, V. 69, n°4, (2001), 2345-2352.

Hackstadt, T., "Biosafety concerns and *Coxiella burnetii*", Trends in Microbiology, V. 4, (1996), 341-342.

Kennerman, E., Rousset, E., Gölcü, E. and Dufour, P., "Seroprevalence of Q fever (coxiellosis) in sheep from the Southern Marmara Region, Turkey", Comparative Immunology, Microbiology and Infectious Diseases, V. 33, no. 1, (2010), 37-45.

Kruszewska, D. and Tylewska-Wierzbanowska, S., "Isolation of *Coxiella burnetii* from bull semen", Research in Veterinary Science, V. 62, (1997), 299-300.

Marrie, T.J., "Q fever. Bacterial Infections of Humans: Epidemiology and Control", Abrutyn E, Brachman PS Edition, Springer, Philadelphia, (2009), 643-660.

Masala, G., Porcu, R., Sanna, G., Chessa, G., Cillara, G., Chisu, V. and Tola, S., "Occurrence, distribution, and role in abortion of *Coxiella burnetii* in sheep and goats in Sardinia, Italy", Veterinary Microbiology, V. 99, (2004), 301-305.

Mazyad, S.A. and Hafez, A.O., "Q Fever (*Coxiella burnetii*) among man and farm animals in North Sinai. Egypt", Journal of Egyptian Society of Parasitology, V. 37, (2007), 135-142.

Muskens, J., van Maanen, C. and Mars, M.H., "Dairy cows with metritis: *Coxiella burnetii* test results in uterine, blood and bulk milk samples", Veterinary Microbiology, V. 147, (2011), 186-191.

Miller, J.D., Curns, A.T. and Thompson, H.A., "A growth study of *Coxiella burnetii* Nine Mile Phase I and Phase II in fibroblasts," FEMS Immunology and Medical Microbiology, V. 42, (2004), 291-297.

Nelder, M.P., Lloyd, J.E., Loftis, A.D. and Revees, W.K., "*Coxiella burnetii* in Wild-caught Filth Flies", Emerging Infectious Diseases, V. 14, no. 8, (2008), 1002-1004.

Niang, M., Parola, P., Tissot-Dupont, H., Baidi, L., Brouqui, P. and Raoult, D., "Prevalence of antibodies to *Rickettsia conorii, Rickettsia africae, Rickettsia typhi* and *Coxiella burnetii* in Mauritania", European Journal of Epidemiology, V. 14, (1998), 816-817.

Palmer, N.C., Kierstead, M., Key, D.W., Williams, J.C., Peacock, M.G. and Vellend, H., "Placentitis and Abortion in Goats and Sheep in

Ontario Caused by *Coxiella burnetii*", Canadian Veterinary Journal, V. 24, no. 2, (1983), 60-61.

Pape, M., Bouzalas, E.G., Koptopoulos, G.S., Mandraveli, K., Arvanitidou-Vagiona, M., Nikolaidis, P. and Alexiou-Daniel, S., "The serological prevalence of *Coxiella burnetii* antibodies in sheep and goats in northern Greece", Clinical Microbiology and Infection, V. 15, no. 2, (2009), 146-147.

Raoult, D., "New rickettsial pathogens", International Journal of Clinical Practice, V. 115, (2000), 79-87.

Raoult, D., Marrie, T.J. and Mege, J.L., "Natural history and pathophysiology of Q fever", Lancet Infectious Diseases, V. 5, (2005), 219-226.

Rey, S., Dennetiere, G. and Rousset, E., "Epidémie de fièvre Q dans la vallée de Chamonix (Haute-Savoie) Juin-septembre 2002", Portail d'Information sur les Etudes Régionales en Observation de la Santé, ARS Rhône-Alpes, (2005), 64p.

Rodolakis, A., "Q fever, state of art: Epidemiology, diagnosis and prophylaxis", Small Ruminant Research, V. 62, (2006), 121-124.
Durand, M.P., "L'excrétion lactée et placentaire de *Coxiella burnetii*, agent de la fièvre Q, chez la vache. Importance and prevention", Bulletin de l'Académie Nationale de Médecine, V. 177, (1993), 935-945.

Rodolakis, A., Berri, M., Héchard, C., Caudron, C., Souriau, A., Bodier, C.C., Blanchard, B., Camuset, P., Devillechaise, P., Natorp, J.C., Vadet, J.P. and Arricau-Bouvery, N., "Comparison of *Coxiella burnetii* shedding in milk of dairy bovine, caprine, and ovine herds", Journal of Diary Science, V. 90, n°12, (2007), 5352-5360.

Rousset, E., "Epidemiology of animal Q fever. Situation en France", Medicine and Infectious Diseases, V. 31, n°2, (2001), 233-246.

Rousset, E., Berri, M., Durand, B., Dufour, P., Prigent, M., Delcroix, T., Touratier, A. and Rodolakis, A., "*Coxiella burnetii* shedding routes and antibody response after outbreaks of Q fever-induced abortion in dairy goat herds", Applied Environmental Microbiology, V. 75, n°2, (2009), 428-433.

Sidi-Boumedine, K., Rousset, E., Hennig, K., Ziller, M., Niemczuck, K., Roest, H.I.J. and Thiéry, R., "Development of harmonised schemes for the monitoring and reporting of Q-fever in animals in the European Union", EFSA Scientific Report on Question No EFSA-Q-2009-00511, (2010), 48 p.

Tissot-Dupont, H., Amadei, M.A.. , Nezri, M. and Raoult D. "Wind in November, Q fever in December", Emerging Infectious Diseases, V. 10, (2004), 1264-1269.

Tissot-Dupont, H., Raoult, D., Brouqui, P., Janbon, F., Peyramond, D., Weiller, P.J., Chicheportiche, C., Nezri, M. and Poirier, R., "Epidemiologic features and clinical presentation of acute Q fever in hospitalized patients: 323 French cases," American Journal of Medicine, V. 93, No. 4, (1992), 427-434.

Thompson, H.A., "Relationship of the physiology and composition of *Coxiella burnetii* to the *Coxiella-host* cell interaction, In Biology of *Rickettsial* Diseases" V. 2, Walker, DH, Edition, Boa Raton, Florida, (1988), 51-78.

Voth D.E. and Heinzen, R.A., "Sustained activation of Akt and Erk1/2 is required for *Coxiella burnetii* antiapoptotic activity," Infection and Immunity, V. 77, no. 1, (2008), 205-213.

Woldehiwet, Z., "Q fever (coxiellosis): epidemiology and pathogenesis", Research in Veterinary Science, V. 77, (2004), 93-100.

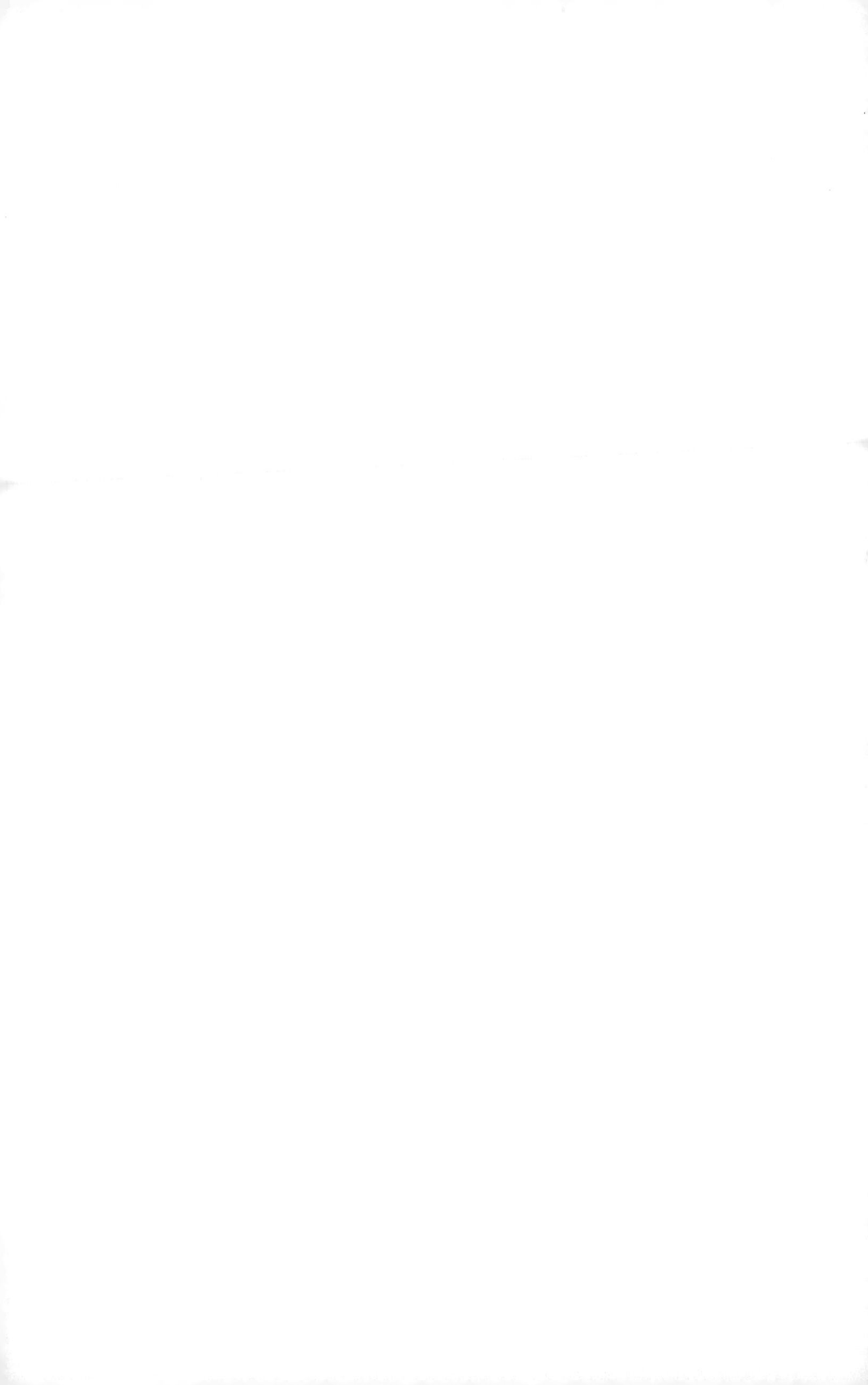

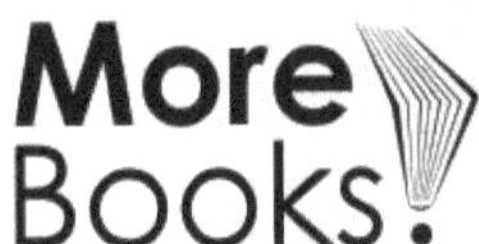

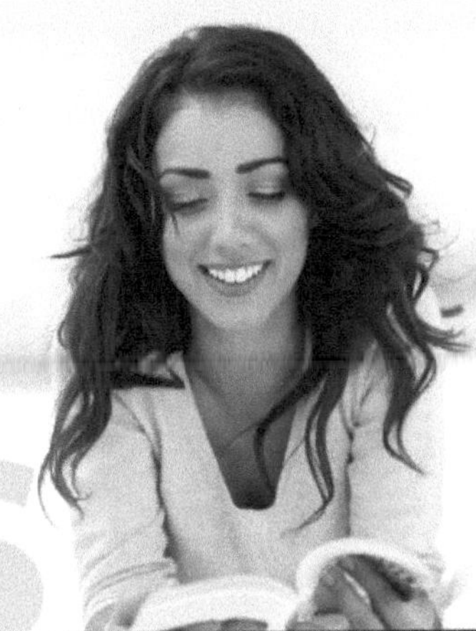

I want morebooks!

Buy your books fast and straightforward online - at one of world's fastest growing online book stores! Environmentally sound due to Print-on-Demand technologies.

Buy your books online at
www.morebooks.shop

Kaufen Sie Ihre Bücher schnell und unkompliziert online – auf einer der am schnellsten wachsenden Buchhandelsplattformen weltweit! Dank Print-On-Demand umwelt- und ressourcenschonend produziert.

Bücher schneller online kaufen
www.morebooks.shop

KS OmniScriptum Publishing
Brivibas gatve 197
LV-1039 Riga, Latvia
Telefax: +371 686 204 55

info@omniscriptum.com
www.omniscriptum.com

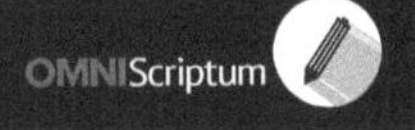

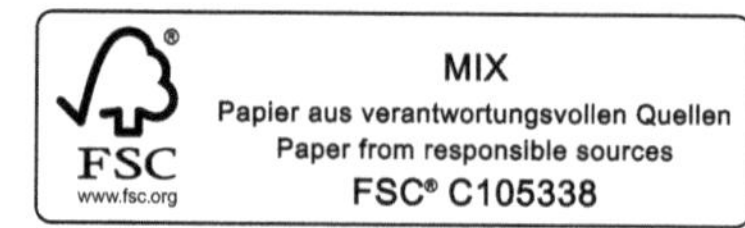